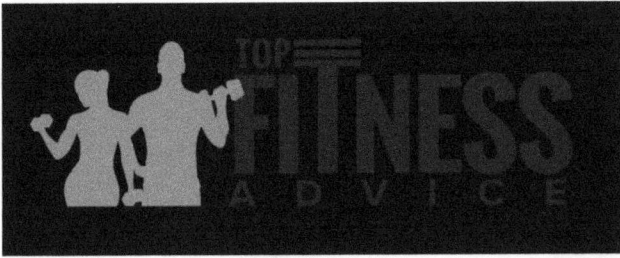

FASTING FOR BEGINNERS

The Easy Way To Fast For Weight Loss (Safely) And Begin Burning Fat, Toning Up & Healing Your Body (And SMASH Food Cravings)

Kayla Bates

ink

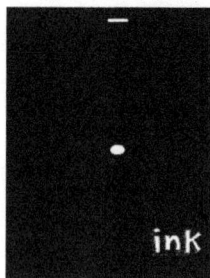

First published in 2017 by Venture Ink Publishing

Requests to the publisher for permission should be addressed to publishing@ventureink.co

For more information about the contents of this book or questions to the author, please contact Kayla Bates at kayla@topfitnessadvice.com

Disclaimer

This book provides wellness management information in an informative and educational manner only, with information that is general in nature and that is not specific to you, the reader. The contents of this book are intended to assist you and other readers in your personal wellness efforts. Consult your physician regarding the applicability of any information provided in this book to you.

Nothing in this book should be construed as personal advice or diagnosis, and must not be used in this manner. The information provided about conditions is general in nature. This information does not cover all possible uses, actions, precautions, side-effects, or interactions of medicines, or medical procedures. The information in this book should not be considered as complete and does not cover all diseases, ailments, physical conditions, or their treatment.

You should consult with your physician before beginning any exercise, weight loss, or health care program. This book should not be used in place of a call or visit to a competent health-care professional. You should consult a health care professional before adopting any of the suggestions in this book or before drawing inferences from it.

Any decision regarding treatment and medication for your condition should be made with the advice and consultation of a qualified health care professional. If you have, or suspect you have, a health-care problem, then you should immediately contact a qualified health care professional for treatment.

No Warranties: The author and publisher don't guarantee or warrant the quality, accuracy, completeness, timeliness, appropriateness or suitability of the information in this book, or of any product or services referenced in this book.

The information in this book is provided on an "as is" basis and the author and publisher make no representations or warranties of any kind with respect to this information. This book may contain inaccuracies, typographical errors, or other errors.

Table of Contents

Disclaimer   3

Who Is This Book For?   7

What Will This Book Teach You?   9

Introduction   11

Chapter 1: What is Fasting?   17

Chapter 2: How Does It Work?   21

Chapter 3: How to Use Intermittent Fasting to Lose Weight 27

Chapter 4: Intermittent Fasting Hacks   41

Chapter 5: Benefits You Can Expect to Experience   45

Chapter 6: Myths Regarding Intermittent Fasting and Weight
Loss   55

Chapter 7: Intermittent Fasting and Exercise   61

Chapter 8: Intermittent Fasting and Muscle Building   65

Chapter 9: How Intermittent Fasting Can Increase Your
Energy   71

Chapter 10: Mistakes to Avoid While Fasting   73

Conclusion   81

Final Words   82

Would you prefer to listen to my book, rather than read it?

Download the audiobook version for free!

If you go to the special link below and sign up to Audible as a new customer, you can get the audiobook version of my book completely free.

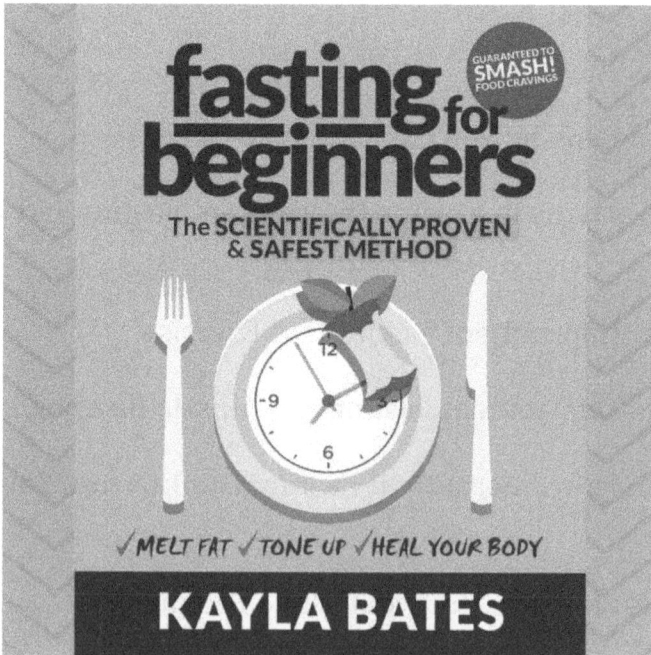

Go here to get your audiobook version for free:

TopFitnessAdvice.com/go/fasting

Who Is This Book For?

Maybe you find that you cannot seem to stop gaining weight, no matter what you try. Perhaps you have lost weight before, but see the scale continually creeping up again, time after time.

Are you ready to step off the rollercoaster ride of weight gain and weight loss? Or continually having to worry whether or not a single slip is going to start you on a downward spiral back to an unhealthy weight?

Scientific research shows that those that consume fewer calories overall actually lead longer and healthier lives. But reducing calorie intake and still eating three full meals a day can be difficult.

You might start out with the best of intentions but, once you start eating and enjoying your meal, it becomes more difficult to stop.

That's where fasting comes in. You can reduce your calorie intact quickly and easily through fasting.

But you have to approach it in the right manner, and this book is going to help you do precisely that.

What Will This Book Teach You?

In this fasting guide, I am going to teach you how to get fasting right so that you lose weight and can keep it off.

But we won't just leave it there. We also look at how vital activity is and how you can use it to improve your results overall.

You will learn why you need to mix fasting with a good dose of common sense and how you can make the most of the experience.

You will learn how to incorporate fasting and exercise into your daily routine.

Introduction

Are you interested in losing weight without having to put in any effort? Does it sound too good to be true?

Okay, you are going to have to put in some effort – you don't get anything worthwhile for nothing – but this program is one of the easiest that you will encounter.

The catch, should you want to know, is that you will be fasting intermittently. You are still going to be able to eat what you like; you are just going to have times in between when you fast.

Needless to say, you can't go nuts with the cheeseburgers or other fast foods, and you will need to eat low-GI carbs, enough protein and generally follow a healthy diet overall.

You will also be drinking a lot of water.

The key to fasting is to follow a reasonably healthy diet most of the time. That way, your fasts can help you build up a real calorie deficit without you needing to extend them for too long.

With fasting, you may fast a maximum of twice a week and not longer than twenty-four hours in any stretch.

How Intermittent Fasting Works

By fasting, you reduce the number of calories that you have consumed for one particular week. By fasting twice a week, you are able to reduce overall consumption per week by about 5000 calories. This roughly translates to 700 calories daily.

The fasting also affects the hormones in your body, allowing the body to reach optimum levels by reducing the amount of insulin in the blood. Your body is primed to start using its fat stores to make up for the energy lost when fasting.

Twenty-Four Hours Without Food

I am going to be straight with you; this is not going to be easy to adjust to. Time your fasts to start just before bedtime – that helps because you are less likely to feel hungry during the morning if you skip breakfast.

So, if you work regular offices hours, have your last meal by 6 o'clock on Tuesday night. Get to bed early and prepare for the next day.

Because you are going to save time on preparing and eating breakfast and lunch, you have time to other things. Take advantage by getting in a nice walk, away from where everyone else is eating.

It will go by quite quickly but if you start feeling hungry, try drinking some cold water. If the pangs are really bad, have some gum without sugar in it.

Are You ALWAYS Hungry When You Try to Lose Weight?

Discover How to STOP Starving Yourself & Lose Weight FASTER By Eating MORE Food!

For this month only, you can get Kayla's best-selling & most popular book absolutely free – *The Ultimate Guide to Healthy Eating & Losing Weight Without Starving Yourself!*

Get Your FREE Copy Here:
TopFitnessAdvice.com/Book

Discover how you can **start eating MORE food** and see weight loss results faster than ever before. Learn about the 10 most powerful fat-burning foods and how they boost the rate that your body burns fat. And last but not least, finally put an end to your emotional or "bored" eating habits. With this book, readers were able to significantly improve their weight loss results. So, it's highly recommended that you get this book, especially while it's free!

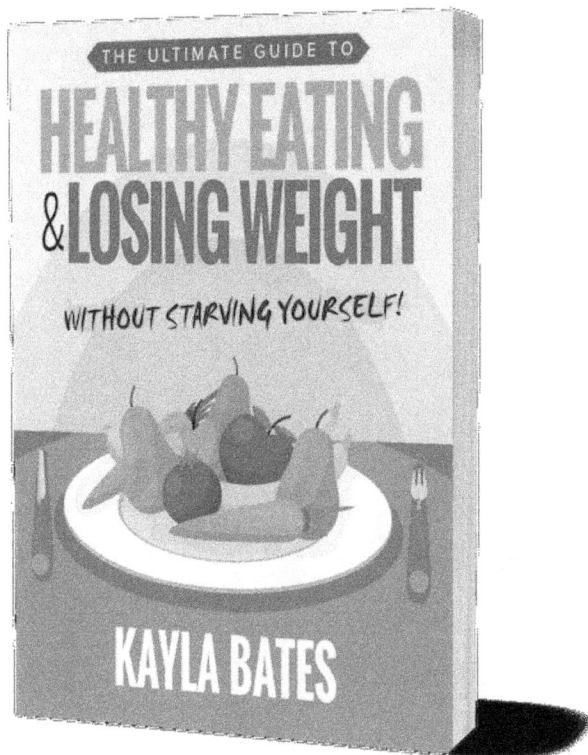

Get Your FREE Copy Here:

TopFitnessAdvice.com/Book

Chapter 1

What is Fasting?

Fasting intermittently means that you alternate between eating and not eating. This often means that only water passes your lips when you are fasting. It's important to keep up your water intake to prevent dehydration.

The amount of time you fast for depends on what you want to accomplish.

Alternate Day Fasting is one sort of fasting that is very popular. You fast for a twenty-four-hour period and then are able to eat what you like for the following twenty-four hours.

This is just one type of fast and it does not appeal to everyone. Here are some others that you might consider:

- Fast for twenty hours out of twenty-four.
- Fast for nineteen hours out of twenty-four.
- Fast for sixteen hours out of twenty-four.

Fasting is healthy, as long as it is appropriately approached. You do need to take some precautions, so you do not damage your health:

- Drink enough water and then some. Don't leave it until you are thirsty to drink water. This already means that you have become mildly dehydrated. Water helps to flush your body of toxins that might cause ill-health.

- Speak to your doctor before you try this if you take any kind of medication daily. For some people, like diabetics, the combination and fasting and taking the usual amount of insulin could be fatal.

- The idea is to fast to give your body a break. Not to force it to switch over to starvation mode. If you fast for too long, your body will switch over and start using the proteins in your muscles for energy.

Can You Ramp Up the Effect of Intermittent Fasting?

What is the first food that you are going to eat after you fast? If you're thinking of wolfing down a cheeseburger and fries, hold on there for a minute.

Do yourself a favor and have a fast, healthy snack that you can eat to take the edge off your hunger. It's natural to crave the high-fat and high-carb options – your body wants to make up for lost calories.

And, while these will not have as much of an impact because you have fasted, they are still going to slow your progress.

Ask yourself why you went through the effort of fasting in the first place – was it to feel better, to lose weight, or perhaps to be healthier? Why go through all that if you are just going to set yourself back by tucking into junk food?

Choosing healthy foods to break your fast with provides your body with the nutrients that it craves without all the extra junk. You actually enhance your results.

Try some of these:

- **Fish:** Oily fish, that is. It is packed with Omega-3 fatty acids that are essential to the health of your body and that enable your body to burn its fat stores. The protein will help you feel full for longer.

- **Lean Meat:** Turkey, chicken and ostrich meats are all high in protein and low in fat. It provides you with energy, iron, and carnitine. The carnitine is the critical element here because it helps your body burn more of its fat stores.

- **Dairy:** Dairy has been shown to improve your body's fat-burning capabilities. It also provides calcium and a good source of protein. Both of which are essential when you are building muscles and strengthening your skeletal structure.

- **Whole Grain Foods and Cereals:** In the short-term, you need to get calories in your body to offset the hunger pangs. You will want to choose high-carb options that give you an instant rush of energy. That's a no-no. They may satisfy you initially, but an hour or two later you will just be hungry again.

  It is far better to choose slow releasing, whole grain foods and cereals. You won't get that satisfying blood sugar bump, but you also won't need to worry about sugar crashes. The fiber in these options helps to make you feel full for longer and protects your digestive tract.

- **Nuts and seeds**: These are Mother Nature's own health foods. They have high levels of beneficial fats and also antioxidants and a range of vitamins and nutrients as well. They can help your body keep the levels of harmful LDL cholesterol in check.

- **Fruits and Vegetables:** You need to focus on foods as close to their natural state as possible for the best nutrients. Fruits and vegetables contain all the nutrients and fiber that you need to keep you healthy and well.

The benefit of eating fruits and vegetables as opposed to taking a vitamin supplement is that the fruits and veggies have the nutrients in the correct concentrations for maximum efficacy.

Chapter 2

How Does It Work?

One of the primary reasons that people look for answers about dieting is that they want to change the way they look. They want to lose weight and tone up a bit.

Can intermittent fasting assist you with this? In this chapter, we will explain not only that it does so, but also why it does so.

What's Going on In Your Body?

The first thing to understand is that your body is going to need some time to adjust to fasting. You are changing behaviors that have become entrenched over many years.

Your body is happy with these behaviors; it will resist change. This means that you will have cravings and you might even feel ravenously hungry at first.

This is normal; your body just does not want to change. If you power through these sensations for a few days, they will pass quite quickly. Once your body has gotten itself used to the new way of doing things, you will soon be back to normal again.

Fasting affects the production of hormones and also the way your body sources energy. Without a ready source of food, your body has no choice but to start burning through its fat stores.

As mentioned before, it can be a tricky balance – you want to "starve" just enough so that your body believes there is a temporary shortage of food. This will encourage it to burn the stored fat. If you take it too far, however, you will experience the opposite effect – your body will think that starvation is imminent and protect itself by reducing your metabolism, becoming as energy-efficient as possible and holding on to whatever calories it can get its hands on.

By making use of intermittent fasting, you can strike the right balance. You will eat just enough to satisfy you and to keep your body out of starvation mode but not enough that your body can get all the energy it needs from the food.

And, believe it or not, intermittent fasting is actually more natural for your body than eating three square meals a day. Our ancestors were hunter/ gatherers. This meant that if they did not find or catch their food, they wouldn't eat for the day.

Naturally, this meant that they would go hungry at times. That's why our bodies start laying down fat stores in the first place – it's a survival mechanism to cope with times when food is in short supply.

The main thing that you have to get right is to ensure that your overall caloric intake is lower than usual so that you can lose weight. So, stuffing your face with pizza just after a fast is going to undo the calories that you saved while fasting.

But fasting is more useful than just a weight-loss technique. It also gives our bodies a break. It provides your digestive system with a proper chance to recover from the almost endless onslaught of food that it has become accustomed to receiving.

It is an easy way to cut out bad foods – you will find that the less you eat junk food, the less you end up craving it as well. You also get to set the times that you eat very specifically. This helps to regulate the production of insulin.

This, in turn, can protect you from developing insulin resistance and diabetes. Because you are concentrating on eating foods that release energy more slowly, you are not subjected to the spikes in blood sugar that lead to the inevitable crashes.

The end result is higher levels of energy and more stable energy production. We now know that losing weight is about more than just restricting the number of calories that you take in. That said, you do need to use more calories than you take in if you want to drop a few pounds. Intermittent fasting is an excellent way to do that.

It actually makes it a lot easier. I realize that it won't seem that way initially, but once you get used to, it really is easier. What would you prefer to do – count every calorie that you eat or fast for a few hours every day instead?

So, how does intermittent fasting help you to lose weight?

1. Appetite Control

Our ancestors were not able to stop off at McDonald's or the Seven-Eleven to pick up a snack or a meal. They ate the food that they could find. When there was no food, they went hungry.

Can you remember the last time that you were hungry? Truly hungry, that is?

Intermittent fasting can help you get control of your appetite. You learn to tell if you are really hungry or if the hunger is a coping mechanism.

If Jim from accounting stresses you out on a day that you are fasting, you won't be able to grab a donut to make you feel better. You will have to learn to cope with it another way.

2. Enhancing Your Metabolism

In a clinical study originally published by the American Journal of Clinical Nutrition in the year 2000, researchers at the University of Vienna found that when someone is temporarily deprived of food, more adrenaline is produced to help reduce the energy deficit.

This, in its turn, makes it easier for the body to burn the fat stored in its cells in order to create energy.

Your metabolism when it comes to fat burning is enhanced, and you lose weight. This is true as long as you don't undo your good work by eating junk food on your "off" days.

You can enhance the effect further by working out on a regular basis. However, you do need to tailor your workouts to match your food intake.

What this means for you is that you must schedule moderate exercise for those days that you are fasting. Schedule the more intense workouts for when you actually have some food in your system.

3. Calorie Reduction

You are eating fewer calories overall, and so you are going to lose weight. This is really a no-brainer.

What You Must NOT Do

- **All things in moderation:** That includes fasting. We have gone over this already – you don't want your body to switch to starvation mode and start conserving energy and fat instead of using it.

- **Watch your blood sugar!** Fasting is not for everyone. If you find yourself feeling exceptionally weak or dizzy, you should drink some fruit juice or tea with sugar in it, just to level things out a bit.

- **Consult your doctor first.** If you have a medical condition, you need to check with your doctor before starting this. If you have to inject yourself with insulin, for example, you need to eat regular meals. Some medications are only correctly absorbed if taken with food. Don't take stupid chances with this one.

- **Choose something that suits you.** You might need to change things up a bit until you find the pattern that suits you best. It is essential that this becomes something that is easy for you. The easier it is to maintain, the less the chances that you will give up on it when the going gets tough.

I hope that you are enjoying this book so far, and if you could spare 30 seconds, I would greatly appreciate you leaving a review on Amazon.com.

Chapter 3

How to Use Intermittent Fasting to Lose Weight

I know that this is the section you have wanted to get started on. In this chapter, you are going to find out how you can use intermittent fasting to lose weight.

We will go through some of the very popular protocols used by people to lose weight. Read through them all to see which protocol will fit in with your lifestyle the best. If you find that one protocol doesn't work for you, you also have a few alternatives to try out.

The Lean Gains Protocol

With this protocol, you are not going to eat anything for 14 out of 24 hours. You are allowed to drink coffee that has been artificially sweetened and can have as much water as you like.

The main rule is that you do not eat anything that has calories in it during your fast. What some people do is to chew sugar-free gum to distract themselves, and drink coffee, tea or diet soda to help them feel fuller.

The best time to schedule your fast depends on your personal schedule but do schedule it so that most of it falls into your sleeping hours.

You could, for example, have your last meal before 7 pm and then not eat again until 9 AM the next day. Doing it this way around could be the easiest because you shouldn't feel like you are missing food.

You should be full from eating dinner and will sleep through most of your fast. Most people aren't hungry on waking so shifting breakfast to 9 AM is not a big deal at all.

The most crucial aspect when you talk about losing weight here is to be consistent. Fast every day from 7 PM to 9 AM. That way your body can get used to the fast quickly and knows exactly where its next meal is coming from.

It also fits in well with people who like morning workouts. Many exercise programs suggest it is better to do cardio first thing in the morning before you eat in order to burn the maximum amount of body fat.

If possible, schedule your cardio so that you can, as soon as it is done, have a good breakfast.

The Warrior Diet Protocol

Many years ago, those being trained for the armed services ate just once a day, usually at dinner time. This was to help them cope during wartime when food might have been scarce, or when they had to fight on an empty stomach.

This meant that they went the rest of the day without food and only ate at night.

The Warrior Protocol is based on this system, and proponents believe that the value of the system is that our ancestors would have eaten their meals at night naturally. It's not quite as strict as the armed service's training was, though – you fast for 20 hours out of 24, so you can have dinner and a snack later if you want to.

The idea is to eat at night – this makes it possible to sleep well because your stomach will not be growling. The first few hours after getting up, you probably won't feel that hungry anyway.

The afternoons, initially, are bound to be where you encounter problems with energy and hunger. You can overcome this by drinking coffee and taking in a lot of water.

Dinner also need not be eaten in one sitting. You can choose to fast if you like from 8 PM to 4 PM the next day. You would need to focus on food that packs a good nutritional punch because you are eating a lot less food than you usually would be able to.

This is a good option if you have a problem with constant snacking, but it is difficult to get used to initially.

The Eat-Stop-Eat Protocol

This is suited to those who already follow a reasonably healthy diet but have found that their weight loss efforts have plateaued. With this protocol, the key is moderation, so you can have a couple of pieces of chocolate, but not the whole bar.

This is not the best protocol if you tend to binge eat.

What is nice about this one is that you actually only need to fast either one day or two days a week. You can then eat as usual for the other days.

There is a catch, though – you need to fast for the whole day and that can be difficult to adjust to initially.

Still, you can use the tricks already discussed to help you get through the day – coffee or tea, lots of water and artificially-sweetened soda can help you to feel fuller.

The key here is to stop yourself from eating everything in sight when you finish a fast.

The Fat Loss Forever Diet Protocol

This protocol is excellent if you really cannot bear to give up your junk food. You get to have a cheat day once every week. The downside of this protocol is that you have to fast for 36 hours straight after your cheat day.

For the remaining number of days, you can practice intermittent fasting as you choose. Those that do take part in the "after cheat" fast suggest scheduling it for when you are really busy so that you have something to distract you from the hunger.

When You Should Stop Intermittent Fasting

It is natural for you to feel some transitional side effects when you first start intermittent fasting. If, however, you find that these do not go away within a week or two, it probably means that your body is not adjusting well to the fasting.

Symptoms that might be telling you it is time to stop are:

- Headaches
- Mood swings
- Bloating
- An upset menstrual cycle
- Fatigue

As mentioned earlier, it is natural for these to occur when starting out. If they are persisting, or if they become unbearable, you need to stop fasting and eat normally for about a fortnight.

You can then start easing yourself back into fasting at a slower pace. So, start with the shortest fasting protocol – the Lean Gains Protocol and, instead of fasting every single day, you make it alternate days instead.

How Will It Work?

You can also decide to make the fast twelve hours instead of fourteen, or increase it to fifteen hours a day. Do not exceed fifteen hours on any one day though.

So, you could, if you like, start fasting at 8 PM on Monday night and break your fast at 8 AM on Tuesday. You would eat normally on Tuesday and start your next fast at 8 PM on Wednesday night.

During this period, you will monitor how your body is coping with the fasting. You should bank on fasting like this for a month before you try to increase the number of fasts you do.

After a month, you can try fasting for two days in a row, and then eating normally for the third day. Again, monitor your symptoms. If you find that you are battling to cope, stop fasting for a fortnight and start up with fasting on alternate days again.

If you manage with the alternate day cycle, but battle with more frequent fasts, do not be too stressed out – fasting is not for everyone. Stick to the alternative day schedule, and you will still experience some benefits.

If, however, you were okay with increasing the fasting to two days in a row, carry on like that for a month and then try increasing it to three days on, and one day off. Carry on like this until you are fasting as often as you want to.

If you switch to a more intense fasting schedule and find that your symptoms are too much for you, give it a break for a fortnight and then stick to the previous level again. This will usually mean that you have found the right fasting schedule for you, so no further adjustments should be necessary.

To boost your results, once you have become used to the fasting schedule, you can start to either incorporate exercise or incorporate more exercise. You don't have to go for a five-mile run, just start increasing the time spent exercising or the intensity of the exercise to a level that is a little challenging for you, but not so difficult that you decide to give up completely.

There is one final trick to getting fasting right – you need to drink enough water. Stir 2.5 ml of table salt into a full glass of warm water in the morning and evening and drink that in addition to your usual water intake.

The salt helps to keep the electrolyte balance in your bloodstream up and so can reduce the adverse side effects of fasting. It also enables you to feel fuller.

If Still

If despite doing the gentlest of the gentle or slow cook fast you still experience symptoms of hormonal imbalance and other conditions, don't hesitate to stop it immediately. It may mean that intermittent fasting isn't for you.

At this point, don't worry or feel bad – there are other healthy ways to lose weight too. That being said. However, most women – even those looking to get pregnant – will most probably do well on the slow cook intermittent fasting protocol for as long as they eat healthy foods during the "fasting" period or eating window.

There are different ways in which you can lose weight. Intermittent fasting has become a popular method of fasting in the recent past. This process involves fasting for a short duration of time.

Fasting for short periods of time will help people who consume few calories, and it also helps them in optimizing the hormones that regulate weight gain or loss.

There are different methods of intermittent fasting to choose from, and you can opt for a plan that you feel is best suited for you. As long as you fast carefully and don't exceed your calorie intake or binge on junk food on non-fasting days, you are bound to drop those extra pounds.

Your body stores away energy or calories in the form of body fat. When you don't consume anything, then your body would change several things within itself to make this stored energy available. It is all related to the variations in the activities performed by your central nervous system and also changes in the levels of various vital hormones in your body.

When you fast, there are a few things that would change with your metabolism. The standard of insulin changes when you fast. When you eat, insulin level increases and when you fast it decreases. A small degree of insulin will help in burning away the accumulated fat.

During a fast, Human Growth Hormone or HGH will increase, and this helps in gaining muscle and reducing fat. Fat cells are broken down into norepinephrine, and this helps in the burning down of fatty acids for generating energy.

Despite the widespread belief that consuming five to six small meals is good, short-term fasting helps in burning fat. Some studies suggest that fasting for 48 hours can assist in boosting your metabolism and fasting for more than 48 hours can suppress the same. Short-term fasting can lead to several changes in your body and also the hormones that are produced.

Intermittent fasting will also help you in reducing calorie intake and help you lose weight. The reason intermittent fasting works is that it reduces the number of calories that you are consuming. The different protocols that you will have to follow during the fasting periods make sure that you aren't consuming more calories than those required by your body.

If you follow intermittent fasting for three weeks, you will be able to see a change in your body and would have noticed a significant weight loss as well. With alternate day fasting, you can lose up to one 1.7 pounds every week.

Intermittent fasting will also help you in losing belly fat and will reduce your circumference. These results indeed are very impressive and show that intermittent fasting is a handyuseful tool for assisting you in losing weight.

Intermittent fasting has benefits that go well beyond just losing weight. It helps in improving your metabolism and will also assist you in preventing many chronic diseases while expanding your lifespan.

Although you needn't count calories when you are on an intermittent fasting diet, overall weight loss usually depends on the reduction in the number of calories consumed.

Studies have proven that intermittent fasting and restriction of calories display the same results when compared amongst members belonging to similar groups. Intermittent fasting is indeed a very convenient way of restricting the calories consumed without making any conscious effort of trying to eat less.

Like mentioned in the previous chapter, intermittent fasting not only helps you in losing weight but it will also assist you in holding on to muscle. One of the most prominent side effects of dieting on your body would be the burning of muscle along with fat.

Intermittent fasting can help you shed weight without any or less reduction in the muscle mass in your body. On a diet with just calorie restrictions, your body would start breaking down muscle to fuel itself.

In calorie restriction diets about 25% of the weight loss was muscle mass, and in intermittent fasting diets only 10% of weight loss was associated with muscle mass.

One study was conducted where the participants were all asked to consume the same amount of calories, except they had to do this in just one huge meal given to them in the evening. They not only lost body fat but also increased their muscle build up, along with a host of other beneficial changes in their health.

However, there some limitations when it comes to these studies are conducted, so you should probably reserve judgment initially. When compared to any standard diet you might have tried; intermittent fasting will help you hold onto your muscle mass while burning away all the unnecessary body fat.

If you want to succeed at intermittent fasting, there are certain things that you should keep this in mind, if you have intent to lose weight. You will need to make sure that the food that you are consuming is high in nutrition. You should try eating whole foods whenever possible. You shouldn't forget how important it is to count calories.

Don't eat too "regularly" on your non-fasting days, not so much that you end up compensating for the calories that you didn't consume on your fasting days.

Being consistent is imperative. This rule applies to any weight loss method that you might try. You need to try it for a few weeks at least if you want it to work.

It will take your body a certain amount of time to get accustomed to this new fasting protocol. You need to be consistent with your meal schedule, and over a period, this will become easy.

Most of the intermittent fasting rules also recommend that you take up strength training. It is paramount if you want to burn your body fat while you are still holding onto your muscle mass. During the initial week or two, you needn't bother counting the calories you consume, but after that, you need to be careful.

If you feel like your weight loss has stalled, then you should reconsider your calorie intake. The requisites of intermittent fasting are that you eat a healthy diet and maintain a negative calorie count or deficit if you want to lose weight. You also should be consistent in your diet and don't forget to exercise.

Well, you need to remember that at the end of the day, intermittent fasting is just a tool that you can make use of when you are trying to lose weight. The primary reason for this is the reduction in your calorie intake. There are some advantages necessary hormones have in the body that contributes to the same.

Intermittent fasting is not going to be a good fit for everyone, but it might prove helpful if you try it out. So, try intermittent fasting for a few weeks, and you will be able to see the change for yourself.

Enjoying this book?

Check out my other best sellers!

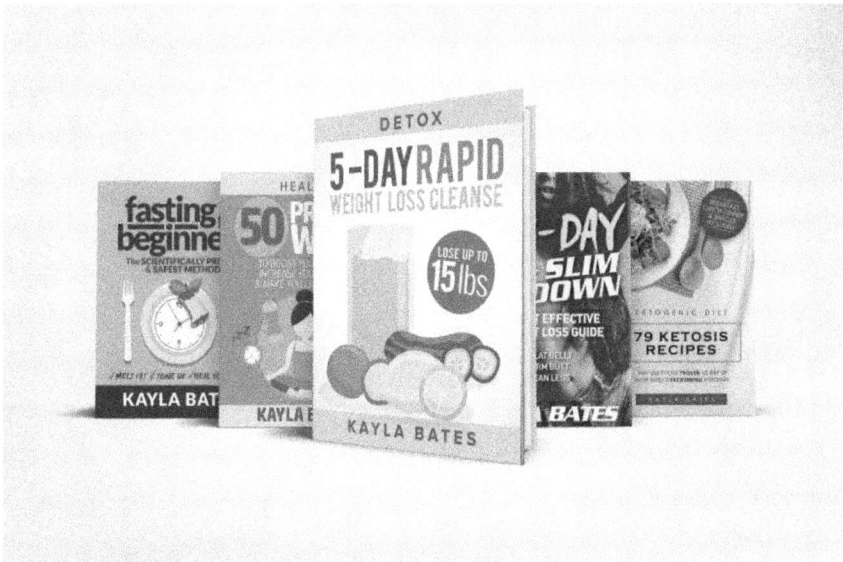

Get your next book on sale here:

TopFitnessAdvice.com/go/Kayla

Chapter 4

Intermittent Fasting Hacks

Intermittent fasting is an easy way to cut calories and drop some extra weight, but there are methods that you can employ to improve your potential results.

In this chapter, we will go through all the hacks that will help you turn your body into a fat-burning superstar.

Get Your Body Moving

There is nothing quite as useful for shaking up your metabolism as exercise, especially when you are following a program of intermittent fasting.

That said, you must time the exercise correctly. While you could, for example, exercise just before you are about to break your fast and eat something, you should never exercise in the middle of your fasting period.

Exercise takes a lot out of your body, and your body requires nutrients to heal itself. If you ignore this, you are likely to feel weak, dizzy and an amplification of any negative side effects of fasting.

Keep your workouts to either right at the end of your fasting period or to those times when you are not fasting.

If you are unfit, or if you are not used to exercising, speak to your medical practitioner before you start training. If you are not sure of how to get started, you should consider getting advice from a personal trainer.

Do be careful to match the level of the exercise intensity to your current fitness level and leave the high-intensity exercises until after you have completed your fasting program entirely. (Especially if you are fasting every day.)

The combination of high-intensity exercise and an intermittent fasting protocol could result in your body being too deficient in nutrients and could harm you physically.

Get the Right Nutrients

Many of us, even those eating three full meals a day, are not getting enough vitamins and minerals in our daily diets. There is a higher risk of nutrient deficiencies developing when you are fasting because of your reduced calorific intake. You can minimize the risk by eating nutrient-dense foods on the days that you are not fasting and choosing foods that are as close to their natural state as possible.

It is also advisable to include a decent daily multi-vitamin and mineral supplement in your daily routine.

Supplement Fiber as Well

A suitable fiber supplement will ensure that you are still getting the correct amount of fiber daily, while also helping you to feel full without adding to your calorie count. It will also help to keep you regular.

The intestines, where our food is sent for further processing to get every last drop of nutrition, and where the benefits of fiber really come to the fore, are 25 feet long.

That's a lot of space for your body to store what will end up as fecal matter. If you don't get enough fiber in your diet, the processing of this fecal matter is slowed down. You could be carrying as much as 15 pounds of it around with you unnecessarily if you eat a diet high in processed foods and low in fiber.

Get enough fiber in your diet and get the digestive process back on track again.

Drink Green Tea

Green tea is high in Theanine, an amino acid that helps to improve metabolism and that can offset the jitters caused by caffeine. Drinking green tea instead of coffee every so often will help to keep you calmly focused and give you a very good dose of antioxidants at the same time.

Theanine has a balancing effect on the nervous system, helping to balance your moods and promote relaxation and a better quality of sleep.

Once again, thank you for reading this book, and I hope you're getting a lot of valuable information. I would greatly appreciate it if you could take 30 seconds to leave me a review for this book on Amazon.com.

Chapter 5

Benefits You Can Expect to Experience

For most people, the primary benefit of this technique is that it helps you drop the extra pounds. The problem is that so many people think of it as a magic pill.

How many times do you read about how, with fasting, you can "eat what you like" on non-fasting days? I am sorry to say that it just doesn't work like that.

Losing weight requires some kind of sacrifice. If it didn't, everyone would be skinny. Something has to give if you want to make a significant change in your body shape.

Fortunately, intermittent fasting can be an excellent way to achieve those changes, as long as you are sensible on the days when you are not fasting.

That doesn't mean that you can never have your favorite junk food again, only that fasting is not a license to eat as much of it as you like. If you start following a healthy eating plan in addition to fasting, you can achieve significant and lasting weight loss.

You can expect to also experience the following.

It Has an Impact on Your Body's "Infrastructure"

When I say infrastructure, I am not talking about your bones and tissue but rather the hormones responsible for regulating everything from how well your cells repair themselves to how your body sources its energy.

Here is some of what to expect when you have not eaten for a few hours:

- Your blood insulin levels drop dramatically, and this has the effect of improving the rate at which your body burns fat.

- The amount of human growth hormone present in the bloodstream can increase fivefold. This, in turn, helps your body to repair itself, increase muscle mass and burn fat.

- The body no longer has to focus on digesting the food, and so it can focus on another task like repairing tissue and cells and removing the waste by-products within them. The body begins to repair its cells and remove waste material that has built up in them

Kick Your Belly Fat for Good

The vast majority of people who do try these protocols do so in order to drop weight.

If you do not change another aspect of your diet except for the introduction of fasting, you will lose weight simply because you are eating less overall. If you couple the fasting with healthy food choices afterward, you are putting yourself on the fast track.

But a very beneficial side effect of losing weight through fasting is that it is very effective at shifting weight from the belly. This is because of the impact on insulin production.

Fasting can help to reverse the symptoms of insulin resistance because of its effect on the production of insulin. Insulin resistance leads to your body packing fat around the middle.

When the insulin resistance is reversed, it is like the fat starts to magically melt away. (It's not an overnight change, but for those who have battled with a jelly belly for years, it will be a noticeable one.)

The lowered insulin levels, combined with more growth hormones and higher levels of norepinephrine mean that your body is more easily able to break down fat and use it for energy.

Fasting in this manner can boost metabolism by as much as 14%, making it even more effortless to burn calories.

Fasting is a two-prong approach – it reduces the number of calories that you consume in the first place and increases the rate at which your body uses calories as well.

According to research, you could lose in the region of 3% to 8% of body weight over a period of 3 to 24 weeks.

You Have Less Risk of Developing Type II Diabetes

Type II Diabetes is considered something of a modern-day epidemic. It usually starts with "simple" insulin resistance. Insulin resistance can be controlled through diet but, if left unchecked, it can develop into Type II Diabetes.

So intermittent fasting can become a useful preventative measure when it comes to Type II Diabetes as well because it can help to regularize your insulin levels.

Research has shown that those who implement this kind of fasting can reduce their fasting blood sugar levels by up to 6%. One study conducted on rats found that intermittent fasting was able to protect the kidneys from damage as a result of diabetes.

I do need to tell you that not all the results are as good. One study found that while men's blood sugar levels did reduce with intermittent fasting, the same was not always true for women. Some women were found to have higher blood sugar levels after intermittent fasting for 22 days. If you are a woman and are concerned about insulin resistance, you really should consult your doctor before starting out.

It Has a Positive Effect on The Hormones

Fasting causes the body to change at a cellular and even molecular level.

Here's how it influences your body:

- **Insulin:** The body is not subjected to floods of insulin. As insulin production becomes more normalized, the body starts to become more sensitive to the insulin it has. It is the high levels of insulin in the body that cause the body to hold onto fat.

- **Human Growth Hormone (HGH):** HGH is boosted during the process, and so your body is better able to repair itself and grow more muscle tissue.

Less Inflammation and Free Radical Damage

When it comes to looking old before your time, free radical damage is your worst enemy. This occurs when the unstable molecules that we call free radicals interfere with the molecules in the cells, protein and even our DNA and damage them.

Fasting improves your body's ability to protect itself against damage from free radicals and also reduces inflammation in the body.

Your Cardiovascular Health Could Benefit

Heart disease causes the most deaths globally at the moment. High LDL cholesterol levels, high blood pressure, high levels of triglycerides, uncontrolled glucose levels and inflammatory markers all put you at a higher risk of developing heart disease.

Research on the effects of fasting in lab animals has shown that fasting can help to reduce all of these risk factors. The results in humans are likely to be similar, but not enough human studies have been done to be sure.

It Encourages Autophagy

When you are fasting, your cells are better able to repair themselves. This includes tasks that they would typically not have the time to undertake like removing waste and excess proteins that start to accumulate in your cells. This is called Autophagy.

It Can Be Used for Weight Maintenance

Fasting is not only useful for those wanting to lose weight but also for those wanting to maintain their goal weight when they do reach it.

It can be used for short periods to give your metabolism a boost if you do start to gain weight again or used on a regular basis if you want to reduce your calorie consumption overall.

Fasting Could Help with Chemo

Chemo makes you feel really awful. One of the worst side effects is the constant nausea. Fasting can help to give you relief from the nausea and so help to reduce the negative side effects that chemo has.

Your Nervous System Benefits

Studies show that fasting intermittently makes it possible to improve the rate of growth of new nerve cells and the level of Brain-Derived Neurotrophic Factor (BDNF) in the blood.

Low levels of BDNF have been linked to increased levels of depression and other issues within the brain. The increased levels of BDNF and the increased nerve cell turnover rate is thought to reduce the risk of having a stroke.

It May Help to Prevent Alzheimer's Disease

Alzheimer's is the leading neurodegenerative disease in the world and is the most common one. Right now, there isn't a cure for this terrible disease, and that means it is more important than ever to look at preventing it in the first place.

Intermittent fasting has been shown to delay the onset of Alzheimer's in some people, and reduce the severity of it in others. It has been shown to defend against another neurodegenerative brain diseases, including Huntington's and Parkinson's.

It Simplifies Your Healthy Lifestyle

It's common knowledge that eating healthy is simple. Still, there's no denying that sticking to healthy meals every day can be incredibly stressful, especially when you take into account the effort to plan and prepare a healthy dish.

Intermittent fasting simplifies this process because it crosses out the need to prepare and cook as much as you used to. For this reason, it is very popular because it makes your life easier while improving your health at the same time.

It May Help to Extend Your Life

It's no secret that a lower calorie intake is a scientifically proven way of prolonging life, and it makes sense from a logical standpoint. When you starve, your body immediately seeks ways of extending your life. The only thing is, why would anyone go into starvation mode just to live longer?

It sure doesn't sound appealing or appetizing in any way. Fortunately, intermittent fasting gives you the benefits of longevity minus the stress of starving. It is because, like calorie restriction, intermittent fasting triggers the exact mechanisms for prolonging life. Longevity is probably one of the most exciting of all the benefits of intermittent fasting.

At this stage, the studies have only been carried out on rats, but they show that, in mice that fasted on alternate days, lifespan was increased by 83% over those that did not fast. The results are not in yet when it comes to human research, but those who are interested in anti-aging measures have adopted intermittent fasting.

Given that intermittent fasting has substantial metabolic benefits, it makes sense that it can help you live a much healthier and longer life. You have heard the phrase that a person with high power has a great responsibility. If you are someone who is going to start intermittent fasting or are someone who has already begun following intermittent fasting, you will need to take care of yourself exceptionally well.

You will need to ensure that you keep yourself healthy; otherwise, you will be harming yourself in ways that will deteriorate your health. I am not trying to scare you off fasting, but asking you to be careful. Let me give you a little information on the detrimental effects of intermittent fasting.

It is Much Easier Than Dieting

Starting and sticking to a diet is one of the hardest things to do for most people. Most dieters fail because they cannot continue with a particular diet for an extended time and end up switching to the wrong foods. The crux of the problem is a behavior change problem as opposed to a nutrition problem.

In this regard, Intermittent fasting takes the upper hand because you get over the conception that you need to eat specific foods (or avoid foods altogether) every time, it becomes amazingly easy to follow.

Studies have proven that intermittent fasting is an effective weight-loss approach in obese adults because the subjects adapted quickly to the intermittent fasting regimen.

Chapter 6

Myths Regarding Intermittent Fasting and Weight Loss

As is the case with diets and nutrition, intermittent fasting too has its share of myths and misconceptions. Read on and do not fall prey to them.

Myth 1: Intermittent fasting will help you lose body fat without undergoing a calorie deficit.

Explanation: When you go without food for extended periods of time, your body starts burning fat as fuel. Fasting also increases your insulin sensitivity levels, which further help in storing less fat.

So, it would seem as if you can lose fat by fasting for a few hours, and build muscle while you are eating.

The problem with this idea is simple — your total caloric intake for the day evens out gradually. If you eat enough during your feed times, you will replace the body fat lost during the fasting state.

Studies have also been conducted which clearly show that there is no substantial evidence to support the theory that intermittent fasting will help you lose your body fat without a calorie deficit. If you wish to lose weight, you need to eat less than you burn.

Myth 2: Intermittent Fasting is detrimental to your health.

Some people believe that fasting is injurious to the health, but that's a wrong preconceived notion. On the contrary, Intermittent fasting has remarkable health benefits, according to recent studies.

From protection against diseases to maintaining good brain health, intermittent fasting positively affects the state of a person's wellbeing. It can also reduce risk factors for heart disease, inflammation, and oxidative stress and can help boost insulin sensitivity.

Myth 3: Intermittent fasting will help you lose body fat and build muscle at the same time.

Explanation: There is almost no scientific evidence that supports this theory. Of course, intermittent fasting does help you lose weight, but that is only during the period where you are in a fasting state.

Moreover, if you adopt the alternate day intermittent fasting method, you will lose less muscle mass than if you choose the daily method.

A complete beginner or novice would do well first to try out the alternate method. That will help him or her to lose body fat and build lean muscle, but not at the same time.

Myth 4: Intermittent fasting is a form of starving.

One of the most common contentions against intermittent fasting is that it's a way of killing and depriving your body of food, which shuts down your metabolism and hinders fat-burning.

Although it's true that prolonged weight loss can decrease the number of calories burned, this is common to weight loss regardless of the method you use. It has not been proven that this is more associated with intermittent fasting than with other weight loss techniques.

As a matter of fact, there is substantial evidence that short-term fasting can improve the rate of metabolism due to a dire surge in norepinephrine levels in the blood.

The bottom line is, fasting, especially for short periods, does not send the body into starvation. Rather, for fasts lasting up to 48 hours, metabolism is boosted by the fast.

Myth 5: Intermittent fasting is a suitable alternative to snacking throughout the day.

Explanation: People will keep telling you different things. Eat six or seven small meals a day. Or eat three large ones and two small ones. Go on a juice only diet. Self-styled dietitians go around advocating these lines to people who are desperate to lose weight.

Nowadays, the trend is reversing, with diet books proclaiming that a large number of small meals per day is not good for the health. But to each his own.

If you find that such an arrangement suits your health requirements, by all means, go for it. Snacking on unhealthy food items in the day is the result of constant hunger brought on by unwise diets.

Intermittent fasting is not a diet. It is simply the rearrangement of your eating schedules. You do get to eat good, wholesome food whenever you sit down for a meal, only the meal frequency changes. Therefore, intermittent fasting is by no means an alternative to snacking.

Myth 6: Intermittent Fasting makes you overeat.

Another unfounded claim about intermittent fasting is that it instigates overeating during eating periods. It is partly correct, as people tend to eat a bit more instinctively during a fast to compensate for the lost calories. However, this doesn't paint a complete picture. For instance, a certain study revealed that subjects who were involved in a whole day's fast ate about 500 additional calories the next day.

During the fast, they burned off about 2400 calories and over-consumed the extra 500 calories the next day. It means that the net reduction in calorie intake was 1900 which is quite substantial for only two days and proves that intermittent fasting helps you lose weight and not gain it.

It is surely one of the most potent tools for weight loss. Implying that intermittent fasting makes you overeat and gain weight could not be further from the truth.

Myth 7: Women should not undergo intermittent fasting.

Explanation: There is some scientific evidence behind the theory that women don't respond as well to fasting as much as men do. One study found that alternate intermittent fasting decreased the glucose tolerance levels in women and their ability to process sugar. It also made them hungrier and more likely to cheat on the schedule. There is no evidence that intermittent fasting is dangerous for women.

Additional studies have shown that while individual women display negative reactions to such a fasting state, it works just fine with other women. It is simply a question of the individual constitution and willpower, and of course, not all nutrition choices, no matter how beneficial, work equally well for everyone.

No matter what your gender, you can, with the right mindset, manufacture an intermittent fasting schedule that works for your body and health needs. Whether you're a woman is not the question at all.

Myth 8: Intermittent Fasting will slow down your metabolism.

Another typical half-truth regarding intermittent fasting is that it ultimately slows down your metabolism. There's a grain of truth in that. When you fast, or your body goes without receiving nourishment, your metabolic rate is lowered as a survival technique to prolong survival. This only happens when you go without food for more than a week.

In fact, one study revealed that in subjects that fasted for three days, there was no slowdown in their metabolism. Plus, Intermittent fasting does not involve fasting for that long, therefore, thinking that your body and metabolism will grind to a standstill is unfounded.

Understandably, this worry is logical because a slower metabolism is every dieter's worst nightmare. However, as already explained, such worries and fears lack basis, because fasting is not dieting.

Others who are considering purchasing this book would love to know what you think. If you could spare a few seconds, they would greatly appreciate reading an honest review from you. Simply visit the page on Amazon.com.

Chapter 7

Intermittent Fasting and Exercise

Ever since the first set of weights in the gym were ever lifted, there has been a debate about whether it's worse or better to use on a stomach with nothing in it.

So many friendships have been severed, marriages destroyed, and lives broken as a result of intense debates on this matter of universal importance!

Alright, exaggeration aside, this is one of the most controversial topics in the world of health and fitness.

In this chapter, you'll settle once and for all this hotly debated topic that has the potential to spark World War III. One of the things we need to first clear is the concept of smaller, more frequent meals when it comes to health and fitness. In particular, that doing so is the best way to rev up the metabolism for burning fat and feeding your muscles.

Contrary to what most people think is true, there are research results that suggest that this just isn't the case.

Another idea or myth to pass away is that working out on an empty stomach will cancel any benefits you may enjoy from working out. Again, some studies have found that that isn't necessarily true.

And lastly, the idea that skipping meals will lead to slower metabolism and stronger desire to eat food, which will consequently lead to weight gain also isn't accurate.

Why do we need to clear those ideas out first? Because those are some of the mindsets or beliefs that aren't consistent with intermittent fasting.

Since intermittent fasting is about, well, fasting; exercising on an empty stomach, eating less frequently and skipping "meals" won't make sense to you and you probably won't believe that exercising while fasting intermittently can be beneficial for you.

Hormonal Optimization

Let me offer you proof that intermittent fasting and working out can coexist and coexist well. Friends, let me offer you: Hugh Jackman. In preparing for his most recent Wolverine movie, Jackman got, pardon the pun, jacked using intermittent fasting.

How's that for proof? How'd that happen you might ask? You see, an empty stomach can help because of hormonal changes inside your body that can foster fat burning and muscle building.

In particular, an empty stomach can improve your sensitivity to insulin and increased natural production of growth hormones, which enable you to grow more muscle mass faster.

Your body produces insulin via the pancreas when you eat, which helps you utilize your foods' nutrient content. Insulin removes blood sugar from your blood and drives them to your fat cells, muscles, and liver for future use.

The problem usually lies when it is too much — and too often — and as a result, your body may become less sensitive to insulin.

Lower insulin sensitivity brings with it a host of other health issues, including inability to lose (or even gain more) body fat and higher risks for cardiovascular diseases and cancer.

Eating less frequently — as is the case when you fast intermittently — minimizes your body's production of insulin and as such, lowers your risk of becoming less and less sensitive to it over time.

The less insulin your body needs to produce, the more vulnerable it becomes to insulin, which helps you burn body fat and lower your risks for diabetes and cardiovascular diseases.

Exercising on an empty stomach also helps your body concoct more of the magical elixir of a hormone called growth hormone or GH, which is important for increasing muscle mass, stronger bones, the ability to burn fat, longevity and improved physical functioning.

Some studies have shown that a man's GH production skyrockets by a mesmerizing 2,000% and a woman's by 1,300% when they fast for 24 hours.

Could you believe those numbers? All by not eating for 24 hours!

And dig this, those studies also showed that as soon as the fast is ended, GH production plummets back down to normal. It is another reason to fast regularly and intermittently — optimal GH production levels.

For men, it's virtually impossible to talk about muscle-building hormones without touching on the big T — testosterone. It's another magical elixir-of-a-hormone that's responsible for muscle building, fat burning, higher energy levels, high libido, and efficiently fighting off depression and heart problems.

Chapter 8

Intermittent Fasting and Muscle Building

Many people have managed to gain weight even while on intermittent fasting, most of which was muscle. It's because intermittent fasting isn't necessarily about cutting down on your total daily caloric intake — though that would be the case if your primary reason for doing it were shedding off body fat — about cutting down on the frequency of eating.

In other words, those who have gained more muscle mass while on intermittent fasting focused on increasing total daily caloric intake during their regular feeding windows. This is not a recommendation to binge eat during your feeding windows. It is simply about choosing healthy, nutritious, and yes, highly caloric foods when you do eat in order to enable your body to gain your desired muscle mass.

The reason why people naturally equate intermittent fasting with fat or weight loss is that of the natural tendency to eat fewer calories when you cut out a meal or two daily. But as I mentioned earlier, intermittent fasting is more about meal frequency and spacing, not total calories.

So, to build muscle, you simply need to consume more calories daily, and you can still do that even if you limit your eating frequency or period. Just consume all your daily caloric needs within the remaining number of meals or food time that you have allotted to yourself.

Apart from having to go on an empty stomach for longer, the other challenge would be to eat more than the usual amount of food per meal or within your eating window. As such, you can still gain muscle, if so desired, while on an intermittent fast.

As a result, more and more people are starting to become curious about intermittent fasting in general and in the different protocols in particular. The choice of which particular protocol to follow all boils down to one's lifestyle and daily schedule.

Some have more time to follow the more time-consuming rules while others have less time available so, the simpler but harder protocols may be just what the nutritionist and trainer ordered for them.

More than the schedule, another aspect of lifestyle is religion. Muslims, for example, are required to fast daily from 5 in the morning to 7 in the evening during Ramadan.

If your reasons for trying out intermittent fasting are one part fitness and health, one part religion or spirituality, rest assured that the two can go hand and hand and there are plenty of fantastic plan choices that should work for you.

Regardless of your circumstances, you can practice intermittent fasting and incorporate a great workout regimen that will enable you to build more muscle and eventually, reduce your overall body fat. It is because muscle cells are metabolically active, i.e., the more of you have, the faster your metabolism becomes.

These guidelines make it possible to build muscle while fasting intermittently:

The Later, the Better

If, as Muslims, you choose a particular period of fasting daily like the Ramadan-prescribed 5 a.m. to 7 p.m. schedule, you'd be well off to schedule your exercise or workout sessions late in the evening or even during the early morning.

Doing so helps you to get your nutrients in before and after working out, especially if you're talking about lifting weights. It gives you, assuming a wake-up call of around 4 o'clock a.m., a six-hour feeding period each day. You can tweak this plan to take every other day off eating as well, especially as you become more experienced and comfortable with intermittent fasting. Do a total fast one day, 6 hour eating period the next.

Post Workout Emphasis

In attempting to build muscle while fasting intermittently, the wisest way for you to apportion your daily calories is by consuming the most significant chunk of your calories during your post-workout meal.

The reason for this is post-workout recovery and calories consumed during the 3-hour golden post-workout window tend to be used more efficiently by the body, e.g., for building muscle instead of being stored as fat.

That being said, you'll need to figure out just how many calories you need to build muscle and consume about 20% of that before exercising or working out. Take in a good mixture of carbs and protein.

Then as soon as you end your workout, consume about 60% of your calories right after your workout and before hitting the sack. If it's too much for you to eat all at once, consider spreading it out over 2 to 3 meals within the next 2 to 4 hours before hitting the sack.

Taking in 60% of your daily caloric requirements may seem too much to take in a relatively short span of time, and frankly, it can be intimidating.

If you find that after several days you're still having trouble doing so, then consider eating foods that are calorie dense, i.e., contain more calories per gram such as dried fruits, red meat, bagels, and raw oats, among others, for you to meet the requirement. Since calorie dense foods have packed significantly more calories, you can eat less regarding volume and still meet your 60% target.

Be sure to select nutritious food. It might seem tempting to choose bacon, cookies, and other junk food in order to pack in a lot of calories in a relatively small amount of time, but you'll not do yourself or your fitness level any favors by making poor decisions. Jerky, nuts, fruit juice with no sugar added. There are a lot of delicious, healthy conscious choices you can make when breaking your fast.

Given that you're going to be consuming the bulk of your daily calories after working out, you'd be better off going higher carb and lower fat than low carbs and high fat. It is because, for post-workout recovery, carbs are better than fat. They are the fastest and easiest energy form to digest and the most natural power source you can provide to your body.

Just take note that low fat doesn't mean any fat. Just keep it to at most 15% of total daily calories. And because fat is the most calorie-dense among the three primary macronutrients at nine calories for every gram as opposed to four calories for each gram of protein and carbs, high-fat foods can be a good way to reduce the volume of food you need without scrimping on calories.

Choose nuts, nut butter, seeds, healthy cuts of meat, and other nutritional sources of fat, and you can enjoy a very decent, high-calorie meal that you might be able to consume in a single sitting.

Eat as Soon as You Wake Up

Lastly, it's best that you eat something right after your natural waking up time when fasting intermittently. If you're sticking to the 5 a.m. to 7 p.m. fasting period Ramadan-style, it means making sure you eat something before 5 a.m.

In particular, go for a slow-digesting protein that can help you feel fuller for longer and help keep your body in an anabolic state, i.e., muscle building state, for longer during the day even without eating. These food items include red meat and cottage cheese, which should make up the remaining 20% of your daily caloric requirements.

While it's not a bad idea to throw in some carbs into the meal, limit the amount so that you get at least 35% of your daily protein-calorie requirements from this meal, which is crucial to maintaining an anabolic state throughout the day. Do this with the goal of consuming only 20% of your total daily caloric requirements for this meal.

Don't Scrimp on the Calories

If you're doing relatively higher intensity or volume workout sessions, just make sure you consume enough calories to power such workouts.

While you can sustain such workouts with low calories and intermittent fasting, it won't be long before you eventually burn out. It's impossible because over time, your glycogen stores will be depleted and your workouts and recovery will be severely compromised. Your substantial gains will cease, and your body will eventually begin to burn through the muscle you already have, leading to muscular atrophy and poorer health overall.

As such, you'll need to learn to eat more food within a smaller period and less eating frequency to ensure you get enough calories to build muscle. It's a good idea to take your time and ease into the change. Start slowly. Over time, you'll adjust to it, and it'll feel natural to you.

I hope you have learned something from this book so far and would greatly appreciate it if you could leave an honest review on Amazon.com.

Chapter 9

How Intermittent Fasting Can Increase Your Energy

So, we've already established the fact that intermittent fasting is capable of helping you lose weight as well as provide a slew of other health benefits. Now, let's tackle energy and how it can help boost yours.

It isn't unusual for people to think that fasting is equal to lower energy levels. After all, we associate food with energy and that the more we eat, the more fuel the body has. However, this is certainly not the case. Eating a lot doesn't always equal a full tank of energy.

In fact, if you've ever observed yourself after eating, you might find that you tend to feel sleepier after a particularly big meal.

How does it help?

First, let's look at the so-called "normal" way of eating. We eat a few times several times each day which also means that our metabolism has a number of different cycles as well, slowly breaking down the carbs from our food and turning it into glucose. It is then used or stored for later use.

After all the glucose has been used or stored, our cognitive abilities and energy levels drop. When this happens, the body sends out a hunger signal—basically beginning the cycle again. This constant increase and decrease in our blood sugar level stresses the metabolism, further resulting in even lower levels of energy and reduced mental performance. Are you familiar with the so-called after lunch lethargy? It is to blame for that.

Now, if you start with the IF program, your body will not have access to the carbs during the fasting period. It makes your body more efficient at using fat as its energy source INSTEAD of carbs. Do the fast frequently, and your body becomes more efficient at this until it practically becomes its natural state.

It is a problem when it comes to weight loss because your body will be turning to STORED FAT for fuel when it comes to producing energy. Slowly but surely, you'll start dropping the pounds without needing to starve yourself. It isn't just weight loss, of course.

Fat is a better source of energy than carbs ever will be—it is capable of providing you with lasting amounts of it without the subsequent crash that you eventually experience with carbs. You'll start feeling energetic and for longer periods of time. Lighter and less tired too. Keep in mind that fats are digested more slowly, and the entire process happens steadily and consistently, giving you a more stable stream of energy.

With that said, do remember that our brain prefers this more than the short bursts of energy that carbs can provide. Our brain uses about ¼ to 1/3 of our overall energy throughout the day, and as such, this stream needs to be consistent for us to maintain a good level of mental performance. It will help us stay alert throughout the day. No more lethargy!

Chapter 10

Mistakes to Avoid While Fasting

Mistake #1: Eating everything in sight

It is one of the most commonly made mistakes. You have to always take in mind, that weight loss with whatever method you choose depends on your calorie balance. You always have to eat less then you burn to force your body to burn its fat to produce energy.

What we do not want is to count calories after every meal like crazy, by looking on every packaging, asking your partner what he or she put into the dinner and focusing only on that.

Still, if you eat only pizza, burger, and cake (sorry for that), you probably won't see any results, because it is too easy to overeat these foods. What you should consider instead are mostly unprocessed food like rice, potatoes, meat, nuts and similar foods.

In general — when you think about healthy food, what comes to your mind? In most cases, this would probably be the right way to eat because we already know what is healthy or not. Salad and chicken vs. Cheese Burger — You decide!

Mistake #2: Thinking all the time about food

It is just like in every other area of your life — if you want to be successful, you have to have a healthy mindset around it.

If you think all the time about food and that you are fasting and that there is such a delicious cake in your refrigerator (sorry again!), then how would you expect not to feel hungry all the time? What you need is a schedule for your day, just do something, distract yourself with things that are not food.

Go to work, waking up a little late, so you have no time for breakfast, go out golfing with friends, and watch an episode of your favorite TV show while drinking a cup of coffee. It is not that hard and will mostly only be in the first days till your body adapts to fasting.

Mistake #3: You start with TOO much motivation

Don't get me wrong; motivation is a beautiful thing to have. With motivation, people can shift mountains, invent electricity and change the whole world. But if you know that everything is a process in which you have to adapt step-by-step then you cannot just go all in, it does not work like that.

You cannot just cut all of your meals to one a day for example. Just take your time and let your body adapt to Intermittent Fasting. Try first one of the "softer" variants like 16/8 and try now and then something like EODD.

Or you can implement once a week the ESE to test your limit. You will see that this way it takes much less effort to adapt Intermittent Fasting to your lifestyle and you will just feel great about it, trust me.

Mistake #4: Being too stressed about the time

This one just goes hand in hand with error #3. Many people think eating one minute or half an hour before the planned feeding window will ruin their diet immediately. They totally forget what Intermittent Fasting was primarily all about. It is about feeling free, being flexible and enjoying a stress less way of dieting throughout your day.

If you planned to eat your first meal at 3 p.m. but feeling so hungry at 2 p.m., then why should you force yourself not to eat?

It just feels wrong! Instead be soft feel free to adapt this diet to **your** lifestyle and **your** feelings. You can just eat an hour earlier and stop eating an hour earlier; it is that simple.

Mistake #5: Focusing on the small aspects

Most people focus too much on little things like a teaspoon of sugar in their coffee instead of just focusing on doing things. They want to know every single detail **before** ever starting their diet, so they never get their results. They want to know whether 20/4 is better than 20.2/3.8 and so on.

Focus on the sum of these details, because many questions are much more important, like what are your goals?

Do you want to gain muscle, or do you want to lose weight? Have in mind that the main thing about Intermittent Fasting are the time windows in which you have to stay in, everything else is too little to know immediately.

Instead, focus on getting started, gain knowledge throughout your journey and get better every day. That's it, that's everything.

Don't forget to share your thoughts on this book by leaving a review on Amazon.com. It takes just a few seconds.

Are You ALWAYS Hungry When You Try to Lose Weight?

Discover How to STOP Starving Yourself & Lose Weight FASTER By Eating MORE Food!

For this month only, you can get Kayla's best-selling & most popular book absolutely free – *The Ultimate Guide to Healthy Eating & Losing Weight Without Starving Yourself!*

Get Your FREE Copy Here:

TopFitnessAdvice.com/Book

Discover how you can **start eating MORE food** and see weight loss results faster than ever before. Learn about the 10 most powerful fat-burning foods and how they boost the rate that your body burns fat. And last but not least, finally put an end to your emotional or "bored" eating habits. With this book, readers were able to significantly improve their weight loss results. So, it's highly recommended that you get this book, especially while it's free!

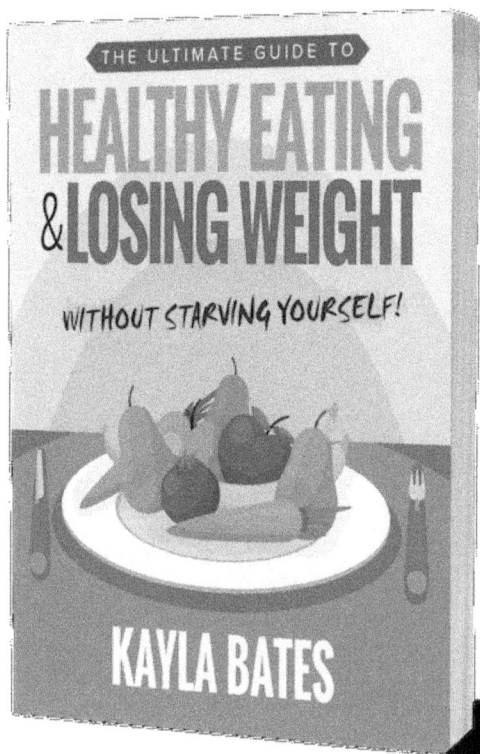

Get Your FREE Copy Here:

TopFitnessAdvice.com/Book

Conclusion

Now that you've finished reading this book, I encourage you to take apply what you've learned here – take action! The value of the information you've learned here is dependent only on your application of them – no application, no value. The best of intentions, after all, is no match for the smallest of deeds.

And when's the best time to act?

It's obviously not yesterday, and it shouldn't be tomorrow – it must be now. The longer you put it off, the higher your risk of not fasting becomes. And there goes your desire to lose weight efficiently and healthily.

So, what are you waiting for?

As the famous sports apparel brand, Nike always says...just do it!

Here's to your healthy and successful weight loss!

Enjoying this book?

Check out my other best sellers!

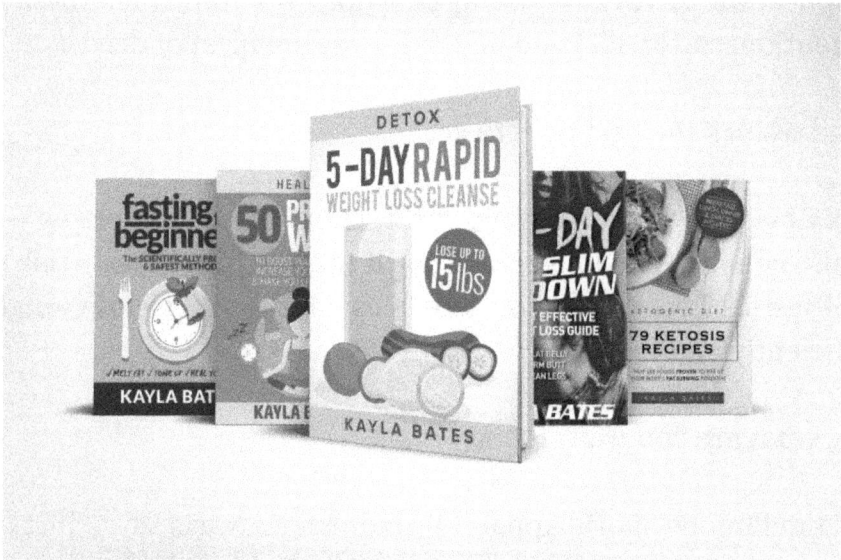

Get your next book on sale here:

TopFitnessAdvice.com/go/Kayla

Final Words

I would like to thank you for purchasing my book and I hope I have been able to help you and educate you on something new.

If you have enjoyed this book and would like to share your positive thoughts, could you please take 30 seconds of your time to go back and give me a review on my Amazon book page.

I greatly appreciate seeing these reviews because it helps me share my hard work.

You can leave me a review on Amazon.com.

Again, thank you and I wish you all the best!

www.ingramcontent.com/pod-product-compliance
Lightning Source LLC
Chambersburg PA
CBHW031205020426
42333CB00013B/801